Table of Contents

Appendicitis Symptoms

Early appendicitis symptoms may be misunderstood as indigestion or gas because mild cramping is common at the beginning. If this feeling lasts for more than 24 hours, and other appendicitis symptoms on the list below begin to appear, it is time to seek medical attention. The most common symptoms of appendicitis in children and adults include:

- Sudden pain that begins at the belly button and shifts to lower right abdomen
- Sudden pain that starts on the lower right side of the abdomen
- Nausea
- Vomiting
- Loss of appetite
- Low-grade fever of around 100 degrees that increases as inflammation and pain increase

- Abdominal bloating

- Constipation

- Diarrhea

- Inability to pass gas

- Right side of the abdomen is tender to the touch

If you are pregnant, appendicitis symptoms may start with pain in the upper abdomen as the appendix shifts slightly higher during pregnancy. Appendicitis in pregnant women is not uncommon; in fact, appendicitis occurs in 1 in 1,500 pregnancies. If you are pregnant and experience any of the symptoms, don't brush them off as early labor or pregnancy related discomfort. Early intervention is key to a healthy pregnancy.

Recognizing appendicitis symptoms in young children is more difficult.

Appendicitis symptoms in young children may include:

- Elevated heart rate
- Fre uent urination

Complaints of stomach pains after moving around, sneezing, coughing or touching their abdomens

If these symptoms appear with an elevated temperature, seek emergency medical attention immediately.

Causes & Risk Factors

While researchers are not sure why appendicitis occurs in some people rather than others, infection, inflammation or obstruction in the appendix or digestive tract seems to be the most common cause. A blockage in the lining of the appendix can cause bacteria to multiply, uickly causing the appendix to become inflamed, swollen and pus-filled. If the appendix bursts, the infection can spread through the abdominal cavity and into the bloodstream.

Recognized risk factors for appendicitis include:

- Age: It most often occurs between the ages of 10 and 30
- Sex: More common in males than females
- Irritable Bowel Syndrome

- Infection in the gastrointestinal tract or elsewhere in the body
- Blunt force trauma to abdomen sustained in a car accident, sporting accident, or fall
- Parasites

Conventional Treatment

Appendicitis is a serious medical condition that re uires emergency medical care. To determine the best course of action, the physician will conduct a physical examination, order blood and urine tests, and often imaging tests like a CT, MRI, or abdominal ultrasound to further understand the condition and appendicitis symptoms you are experiencing. A full medical history will be taken. Also, the medical team will likely ask about digestive symptoms including recent bowel movements.

If the appendix hasn't ruptured, antibiotics will be administered. In addition, 12- to 24-hour monitoring in the hospital may be necessary. But, if the appendix bursts, it will be surgically removed. Most appendectomies today are performed as a laparoscopic procedure, which allows for less pain and scarring and facilitates uicker healing. However, if the appendix has burst and infection is leaking into the abdominal cavity, laparoscopic surgery may not be appropriate.

When the appendix bursts and leaks bacteria and pus into the abdomen, the surgery is more involved as the surgeon must clean the bacteria and pus from the abdomen. After surgery, a tube will remain for a couple of weeks to allow the abscess to continue to drain. Antibiotics will be prescribed to rid the body of the infection. After an appendectomy, most patients are released within a couple of days.

Currently, there is a clinical trial underway by the David Geffen School of Medicine at UCLA to determine whether treating appendicitis (prior to rupture) on an outpatient basis with just antibiotics is safe and effective. Initial results are promising. Researchers anticipate final results in 2021.

16 Natural Ways to Boost Appendicitis Recovery

Follow your surgeon's recommendations for activity, medications and wound care.

Generally, after laparoscopic surgery, you will need to limit activity for three to five days. For an open appendectomy, you must limit activity for 10 to 14 days. Move around slowly and deliberately; avoid carrying or picking up heavy objects. The incision site needs to stay clean and dry.

Practice guided imagery.

According to the Mayo Clinic, after an appendectomy, guided imagery may help to control pain. This can be particularly helpful for children who may experience anxiety, as well as pain, after surgery. Guided meditation is known to relieve anxiety, reduce pain, improve sleep uality and so much more.

Cough carefully.

After an appendectomy, coughing is painful. To prevent some of the pain, apply pressure to your abdomen before you cough. Roll a towel or use a pillow, place it against your abdomen and exert a moderate amount of pressure on it before a cough or sneeze to prevent pain.

Aromatherapy.

An appendectomy is a traumatic physical event, and it takes time to recover. Getting plenty of rest and relaxation after surgery will help you feel better and heal more uickly. To stimulate relaxation, reduce pain, and for better sleep, practice aromatherapy.

Research shows that aromatherapy using lavender essential oil reduces mental stress and anxiety. After a trauma of this nature, children are particularly susceptible to fear and anxiety. Diffusing essential oils can help to relieve these emotions.

For pain, there are a broad range of studies that show aromatherapy aids in the reduction of pain and may have a long-term effect on pain reduction for burn patients, rheumatoid arthritis, during labor, and for those living with chronic pain. A couple of these studies specifically identified lavender essential oil or a combination of rose and lavender oils, while other studies didn't specify the essential oil tested.

Homeopathic arnica 6x.

Known for its anti-inflammatory and pain relieving properties, arnica may also decrease swelling after the surgery. Use as directed for two weeks following surgery.

Support healthy liver function.

After appendicitis, supporting liver function is essential. Anesthetics used during surgery can cause a decrease in liver function, allowing toxic substances to build up. In the weeks after an appendectomy, avoid consuming too much caffeine and alcohol, as well as conventionally farmed fruits, vegetables and meats. Focus on fresh, organic produce, grass-fed organic meat, and wild-caught fish like salmon.

Boost immune system health.

Avoiding an infection after an appendectomy, particularly if the appendix ruptured and leaked bacteria and pus into the abdominal cavity, is a must.

The best way to guard against infection is to ensure your immune system is performing optimally. Practice the best tips to boost your immune system including adding high- uality supplements like ginger, ginseng, vitamin D, and others to your healing plan.

The appendix is a part of the digestive tract, so you may experience some new gastrointestinal symptoms as you heal. Rely on a healthy diet and avoid any processed foods and any foods that you are sensitive to, including gluten and conventional dairy. Eat small, nutrient-dense meals in the weeks following surgery, and enjoy my favorite gut-healing smoothie recipe, sure to please kids and adults alike.

Bromelain.

In a small study conducted by researchers at the University of Texas's Advanced Wound Healing and

Tissue Regeneration Laboratory, a supplement containing vitamin C, grape seed extract, rutin and bromelain supported faster healing, and participants experienced less redness and swelling.

Bromelain, an enzyme found in pineapple, demonstrates incredible proven health and therapeutic benefits including helping to prevent cancer, cardiovascular disease and diabetes. After surgery, take 1,000 milligrams of a high- uality bromelain supplement three times each day to spur healing.

Vitamin C.

Vitamin C helps the body to metabolize anesthetics used during surgery and may help to speed healing, according to researchers from Gundersen Lutheran Medical Center. Dr. Michael A. Fiorillow, MD, a leading plastic surgeon, recommends 2,000 milligrams a day of a high- uality vitamin C supplement to anyone with an open wound as it helps the wound heal faster.

In addition, make a point to consume organic vitamin C-rich foods like guava, oranges, red or green peppers and papaya. Vitamin C boosts the immune system and helps to improve mineral absorption, which is key when recovering from surgery.

Vitamin A.

If you have Crohn's disease, are a vegan, have problems with your pancreas, or have cystic fibrosis, you may be deficient in vitamin A. Vitamin A deficiency can make you more susceptible to developing an infection, which can be incredibly dangerous after surgery and trauma.

The recommended daily allowance for vitamin A is as follows:

Children:

1–3 years old: 300 micrograms/day

4–8 years old: 400micrograms/day

9–13 years old: 600micrograms/day

Adult Females:

14 years old and up: 700 micrograms/day

When pregnant: 750–770 micrograms/day

When breastfeeding: 1,200–1,300 micrograms/day

Adult Males:

14 years old and up: 900 micrograms/day

Also, add plenty of vitamin A-rich foods like wild-caught tuna, carrots, sweet potatoes and leafy greens to your diet to help boost immune system function when recovering from appendicitis.

Zinc.

Even a mild zinc deficiency can interfere with healing. According to Boston University School of Medicine, an increased consumption of vitamin A, vitamin E and zinc may influence wound healing rates. Enjoy zinc-rich foods during your healing like grass-fed beef and lamb, pumpkin seeds, chickpeas and even cocoa powder.

Arginine & omega-3.

A study conducted by Shriners Hospitals for Children and University of Cincinnati Medical Center found that the combination of arginine and omega-3 fatty acids reduced surgical site infections by 50 percent, significantly reducing hospital and ICU stays.

In the study, 10 grams of arginine were given, along with a customized dose of omega-3, based on 3.5 percent of energy for each patient. As a precaution, arginine should not be given if the patient is septic, or for those who have high blood pressure.

Glutamine

An essential amino acid, glutamine supports gastrointestinal health. Also, research shows that it reduces the risk of infection after surgery or injury, according to researchers from Brigham and Women's Hospital at Harvard Medical School. During recovery, take between 2 and 5 grams of glutamine twice a day, along with a high-quality vitamin B12 supplement for best results.

Probiotics.

The anesthetics from the surgery and the antibiotics harm the gut's natural healthy bacterial balance. To rebuild the healthy bacteria, take a high- uality probiotic supplement that provides at least 50 billion CFU per serving. In addition, add probiotic-rich foods to your diet in the following weeks, including kefir, yogurt, sauerkraut and apple cider vinegar.

Coconut Oil.

To prevent significant scarring, once the stitches or the staples have been removed, gently massage coconut oil around the scar. It will help to nourish the skin and help to thwart any lingering fungi, bacteria or viruses lurking on the skin.

Enjoy a healthy, clean diet.

The appendix is part of the digestive system, so during recovery, a healthy, clean diet is essential. Dr. Elson M. Haas, MD, founder and director of Preventive Medical Center of Marin in San Rafael, California says that a diet after surgery should be light, not greasy, and easy to digest. Focus on nutrient-dense protein powders, bone broth and organic foods.

Precautions

If the appendix ruptures, the infection and bacteria can spread throughout the abdomen causing peritonitis; this can be life-threatening. Take appendicitis symptoms seriously and seek medical intervention uickly.

After an appendectomy, seek medical attention if you experience fever, chills, bleeding or drainage from the incision site, vomiting, loss of appetite, coughing, shortness of breath, cramping, no bowel movement for two days or longer, or diarrhea for three or more days

6 Tips for Recovering From an Appendectomy

First, Emergency Surgery. But Then What?

Appendectomy is one of the top reasons for emergency general surgery in the United States. An emergency appendectomy is the standard treatment for appendicitis—inflammation of the appendix, a small pouch that extends from your colon on the lower right side of your abdomen. Removing the appendix is the only way to protect you from the dangerous infection that could develop if your appendix bursts. Whether your appendectomy surgery is open (with a large incision through the abdomen) or laparoscopic (with 1 to 3 small incisions), it's important to take these six steps for a smooth and complete recovery.

1. **Allow yourself to rest.**

When a person has surgery, the body's natural response is to throw the brakes on regular activity so it can focus on uninterrupted healing. That means you can expect to sleep much more than usual for at least the first week or so following surgery. This period of decreased physical activity is important, especially with abdominal surgery (either open or laparoscopic). That's because your surgeon had to cut through the external muscles you can see as well as the innermost layer of the abdominal wall that keeps your internal organs in place. If you resume activities before the inner layer heals, a hernia may develop, in which part of your intestine s ueezes out of the abdominal cavity. This may lead to the need for more abdominal surgery to repair the hernia.

2. Follow your doctor's instructions.

Your doctor will give you specific homecare instructions when you leave the hospital. These instructions will most likely cover wound care, any dietary restrictions, and signs of possible complications specifically related to your surgery. The instructions should also spell out any limits your doctor is placing on your activities while you heal. Expect limits to be placed on how much weight you can lift and for how long. Each surgeon's preferences vary but, in general, the more closely you follow the homecare instructions, the smoother your recovery will be.

3. **Manage your pain.**

Being in pain puts extra stress on your body and can slow the healing process. Your doctor's homecare instructions will likely include suggestions about how to manage surgical pain. Follow the instructions about pain medications exactly. In general, you want to take the smallest possible dose for the shortest possible time while still getting relief. Call your doctor if your pain medications aren't helping. Tip: You can help reduce pain by placing a pillow over your abdomen and applying gentle pressure before you cough, laugh or move.

4. **Increase your activities gradually.**

Rest is important, but so is gentle activity. When you're ready, start slowly and increase your activity as you feel up to it. Short walks, even just around the house, are a great way to start and help protect you from developing pneumonia or blood clots. An added bonus: Being up and about will encourage your digestive system to return to normal sooner. Constipation can be very uncomfortable, so walk when you can, get plenty to drink, and take stool softeners if your doctor recommends them.

5. **Know the signs of infection.**

Infection is the biggest risk following appendectomy. You can minimize this risk by following your doctor's wound care instructions carefully. You should also watch for signs of infection, which include redness and swelling around the incision, fever above 101 degrees Fahrenheit, chills, vomiting, loss of appetite, stomach cramps and diarrhea. Call your doctor if you are concerned about any symptoms you experience.

6. Ease back into regular life.

Your surgeon will typically want to check your progress at a follow-up visit about 2 to 3 weeks after surgery. You may be tempted to skip the visit if you're feeling better, but don't. You want to make sure everything is healing well, and discuss how long any activity restrictions must remain in place. Adults may have returned to work by the time of the follow-up visit, but children may need a doctor's clearance to return to school or physical activities. Appendectomy is considered emergency surgery, but it's also one of the most common abdominal surgeries performed in the United States, so by the time you're a few weeks out of surgery, life should be back to normal—minus one appendix, that is.

1. 12 Bean Soup

Ingredients:

2 c. 12-bean soup mix*

1 ham bone (optional)

4 T. BBQ sauce

1 chopped onion (can use food storage substitution, see chart)

1 T. sugar

1 small clove garlic

3 stalks celery, diced (can use food storage substitution, see chart)

¼ tsp. lemon pepper

2 carrots, diced (can use food storage substitution, see chart)

2 T. ketchup

28 oz. can whole tomatoes

¼ tsp. salt and ginger

1 pinch red pepper flakes

You can buy this as a mix or make your own with legumes in your food storage

Directions:

Wash 2 cups of bean mix. Soak in a large pot overnight. Drain. Add 8 cups water, ham bone, 1 tsp. salt, and ¼ tsp. ginger. Bring to a boil and cook until beans are tender (about 1 hour). Add remaining ingredients. Bring to a boil. Simmer 2 ½ to 3 hours. Stir and add water as needed. For more zest, double all spices.

2. **Baked Oatmeal**

Ingredients:

2 c. uick oats

½ c. brown sugar

⅓ c. raisins

1 T. chopped pecans

1 tsp. baking powder

1 ½ c. skim milk (can use food storage substitution, see chart)

½ c. applesauce

2 T. butter, melted

1 large egg, beaten (can use food storage substitution, see chart)

Directions:

Preheat the oven to 375 degrees. Combine the first five ingredients in a medium bowl. If using dry milk and dry eggs, add those powders to the dry ingredients. Combine the milk (or water), applesauce, butter, and egg (or water) in a separate bowl. Add wet mixture to dry ingredients; stir well. Pour into a greased 8" s uare baking dish. Bake for

3. Basic Meatball Recip

Ingredients:

1 lb ground beef

⅓ c. milk

½ c. fine dry bread crumbs

¼ c. dehydrated onion

1 egg

1 tsp. salt

Directions:

Mix all ingredients together. Shape into meatballs (it's easiest with a melon or ice cream scoop) and put on a rack with a pan underneath. Cover the pan with tinfoil to save on clean-up time. Bake at 425 for about 15 minutes. This recipe freezes well.

4. Beach Street Lemon Chicken Linguine

Ingredients:

1 lb linguine (or fettuccine)

2 T. olive oil

Zest from one lemon

Juice from one lemon

½ c. chopped green onion (can use food storage substitution, see chart)

¼ c. chopped fresh parsley (can use food storage substitution, see chart)

Salt and freshly ground pepper

Parmesan cheese

Marinade:

½ c. olive oil

2 cloves garlic, whole

2 T. cajun seasoning

2 T. lemon juice

2 T. minced parsley (can use food storage substitution, see chart)

1 T. brown sugar

2 T. soy sauce

2 chicken breasts, sliced (can use food storage substitution, see chart)

Directions:

Combine the marinade ingredients in a Ziploc bag. Add sliced chicken. Refrigerate 1-12 hours. Cook marinated chicken with the marinade sauce in a large saute pan.

Cook linguini in boiling water. Drain noodles. Combine juice of one lemon, zest, olive oil green onions, and fresh parsley together to the noodles. Add in chicken and salt and pepper. Toss in parmesan cheese to taste and serve warm. *Recipe from Deals to Meals

5. Best Rice Krispie S uares

Ingredients:

½ c. white sugar

1 c. corn syrup

¾ c. peanut butter

2 c. Rice Krispies

4 c. Corn Flakes

Directions:

Use a large pot and stir together first three ingredients until melted & smooth. Do not overcook. Once you have a nice mixture, still in the cereal. You will want your pot to be big enough. Spread in a 9×13 pan.

6. Best Whole Wheat Bread Recipe

Ingredients:

7 c. whole wheat flour (fresh ground is best)

⅔ c. vital wheat gluten

2 ½ T. instant yeast

5 c. hot water (120-130 F)

2 T. salt

⅔ c. oil

⅔ c. honey

2 ½ T. bottled lemon juice

5 c. whole wheat flour

Directions:

Mix together the first three ingredients in your mixer with a dough hook. Add water all at once and mix for 1 minute; cover and let rest for 10 minutes (this is called sponging). Add salt, oil, honey, and lemon juice and beat for 1 minute.

Add last flour, 1 cup at a time, beating between each cup. Beat for about 6-10 minutes until dough pulls away from the sides of the bowl. This makes very soft dough. Spray counter with Pam and take dough out of the bowl. Do NOT flour your counter, this will add dryness you don't want in the bread. You basically want your dough to feel a "little" sticky. Separate dough. Form into loaves and place in bread pans. Let rise until double in size. Bake at 350 for 22-30 mins or until browned. Makes 6 small to medium loaves.

7. Blackberry Pie

Ingredients

Pie Crust:

2 c. flour

1 T. salt

¾ c. butter flavored shortening

1 T. egg powder

¾ c. cold water

Blackberry Filling:

5-6 c. freeze-dried blackberries, rehydrated and

drained

1 T. lemon juice

¾ c. white sugar

3 T. corn starch

⅛ tsp. cinnamon

Instructions:

Combine flour and salt. Cut in the shortening until the mixture is crumbly. Combine the egg powder and water. Add to the flour mix and stir until dough is formed. This makes avery soft, sticky dough. Split into two pieces. Refrigerate for an hour for easier rolling. Roll out half the dough on a floured surface and place into a 9" pie crust. Put back in fridge while you prepared the filling. For the filling, after the blackberries are hydrated and drained, mix with lemon juice. Combine the other ingredients in a bowl and pour in the blackberries. Mix it all around and pour into the pie shell. Roll out the other half of the dough and cut it into 1 inch slices. Lay in a criss-cross pattern. Mix up a tiny bit of powdered milk with about twice the amount of powder as it normally calls for. Brush over top of the crust and then sprinkle with white sugar. Cover the edges with tinfoil and bake at 425 for about 30 minutes or until the crust is golden brown and delicious.

8. Blender Wheat Pancakes

Ingredients:

1 c. milk (can use food storage substitution, see chart)

1 c. wheat kernels, whole & uncooked

2 eggs (can use food storage substitution, see chart)

2 tsp. baking powder

1 ½ tsp. salt

2 T. oil

2 T. honey or sugar

Directions

Put milk and wheat kernels in blender. Blend on highest speed for 4 or 5 minutes or until batter is smooth. Add eggs, oil, baking powder, salt and honey or sugar to above batter. Blend on low. Pour out batter into pancakes from the actual blender jar onto a hot greased or Pam prepared griddle or large frying pan. Cook; flipping pancakes when bubbles pop and create holes.

9. Brown Sugar

Ingredients:

1 c. white sugar

1-2 T. molasses

Directions:

Use this recipe if you are out of brown sugar. This brown sugar can be made right before use, so there is no worry of having your brown sugar harden and become unusable. Mix sugar and molasses together. Depending on how dark you want the sugar, add more or less molasses.

10. Buttermilk Cornbread

Ingredients:

½ c. butter

⅔ c. white sugar

2 eggs (can use food storage substitution, see chart)

1 c. buttermilk (can use food storage substitution, see chart)

½ tsp. baking soda

1 c. cornmeal (grind your own with popcorn kernels)

1 c. all-purpose flour (works with whole wheat too)

½ tsp. salt

Directions:

Preheat oven to 375 degrees. Grease an 8 inch s uare pan. In a large bowl combine melted butter and white sugar. Quickly add eggs and beat until well blended.

Combine buttermilk with baking soda and stir into mixture in pan. Stir in cornmeal, flour, and salt until well blended and few lumps remain. Pour batter into the prepared pan.

Bake in the preheated oven for 25 to 30 minutes, or until a toothpick inserted in the center comes out clean.

11. Cheesy Ritzy Potatoes

Ingredients:

4 c. freeze-dried potato dices

⅓ c. dehydrated onion flakes

2 cans cream of chicken soup

1 c. sour cream powder, hydrated

¾ c. freeze-dried cheddar cheese

½ c. powdered butter, hydrated

2 tubes ritz crackers crushed

Directions:

Preheat your oven to 350 degrees. Soak your potato dices and dehydrated onions in warm water. In a separate bowl, soak your freeze-dried cheddar cheese. While they are soaking, mix up your sour cream powder with water. Stir in your cream of chicken soup. Drain your potatoes and pour them into a 9×13 casserole dish. Drain the rehydrated cheese and add it to the cream mixture. Pour the cream mixture over top of the potatoes and stir together well. In a small bowl mix up your powdered butter. Add the crushed ritz and mix well. Cover the dish with tinfoil and bake for 30-40 minutes.

You can remove the foil for the least 5 minutes to get the topping more browned. While this works with powdered butter it's better and easier with regular melted butter

12. Chicken Barley Chili

Ingredients:

1 (14.5 oz) can Italian diced tomatoes

1 (16 oz) jar/can Salsa or tomato sauce

1 (14.5 oz) chicken broth

1 c. Quaker Quick Barley

3 c. water

1 T. chili powder

1 tsp. cumin

1 (15 oz) can black beans, drained and rinsed

1 (15 oz) can corn, drained

1 ½ lbs boiled chicken breasts in chunks (can use food storage substitution, see chart)

Cheddar cheese, sour cream, tortilla chips (optional)

Directions:

In a large pot, combine the first 7 ingredients. Bring to a boil, cover and reduce heat to low. Simmer for 20 minutes, stirring occasionally. Meanwhile boil the chicken in a separate pan. Add beans, corn, and chicken to large pot. Cook on high until chili comes to a boil. Cover and reduce heat to low. Simmer for another 5-10 minutes or until barley is tender. If desired, top with shredded cheese, sour cream, and tortilla chips.

Makes a huge batch!

13. Chocolate Cake

Ingredients:

3 c. sifted flour

2 c. sugar

2 tsp. baking soda

1 tsp. salt

⅓ c. dark chocolate cocoa powder

2 tsp. white vinegar

2 tsp. vanilla

¾ c. canola oil

2 c. water

Frosting ingredients (see below)

Directions:

Pre-heat oven to 350 degrees. Put all dry ingredients into a large bowl and sift together. Mix all the wet into one bowl then add to dry ingredients. This is a really wet batter and there may be a few lumps. Pour into a 13 x 9 ungreased pan. Bake for approximately 40 minutes at 350. (Reduce oven temperature to 325 degrees and increase cook time to 45 minutes for a glass pan).

Frosting:

Set aside 1 cup chocolate chips and 2 handfuls of marshmallows. In a sauce pan add:

1 cup sugar, ¼ cup butter, ¼ cup milk. Stir occasionally on a medium heat until it comes to a boil. Do not boil. Remove from burner. Stir in 1 cup chocolate chips and 2 handful's of marshmallows until melted into frosting. Frost cake.

14. Chow Mein Casserole

Ingredients:

1 lb hamburger (can use food storage substitution, see chart)

½ an onion chopped (can use food storage substitution, see chart)

½ c. rice, cooked

2 cans cream of chicken soup (use Cream of Chicken Soup recipe included)

1 ½ c. hot water (if using bean flour Cream of Chicken Soup, skip the water)

⅛ c. soy sauce

¼ tsp. ground pepper

½ can chow mein noodles (about 3 oz)

Directions:

Preheat oven to 350º. Mix all ingredients together (except chow mein noodles). Bake in serving bowl covered with foil for 45 minutes. Take off cover. Pour 3 oz. (½ can) of chow mein noodles over top. Cook uncovered for 15 more minutes. Let set for 5-10 minutes after cooking to thicken.

15. Cookie Clay Dough

Ingredients:

½ c. sugar

½ c. brown sugar, firmly packed

½ c. butter (1 cube)

1 tsp. vanilla

1 egg (can use food storage substitution, see chart)

2 c. whole wheat flour

1 extra large egg (can use food storage substitution, see chart)

1 tsp. baking powder

½ tsp. salt

½ tsp. cinnamon

Directions:

Cream together first 5 ingredients with a mixer.

In a separate bowl combine all dry ingredients.

Slowly add to the creamy mixture until it reaches the consistency of PlayDoh. Give the Cookie Clay Dough to your kids and let them make shapes, letters out of it. They can use it like they would use regular Play-Doh. Once they are finished, put all of the shapes on a cookie sheet and bake at 350 degrees for 10-15 minutes. *Recipe from

16. Corn Dog Muffins

Ingredients:

1 ½ c. cornmeal (about 1 c. fresh ground popcorn)

2 ½ c. flour (about 2 c. fresh ground wheat)

½ c. white sugar

¼ c. brown sugar

4 tsp. baking powder

1 tsp. salt

2 eggs (can use food storage substitution, see chart)

2 c. milk (can use food storage substitution, see chart)

8 oz. shredded cheddar cheese

6 hot dogs cut in thirds

Directions:

Preheat oven to 400 degrees. Mix dry ingredients in large bowl. Beat eggs and milk in a separate bowl. Add to dry mix and add cheese just until moistened. Spoon mixture into muffin tins until ⅔ full. Add 1 hot dog chunk to each muffin. Bake for 14-18 minutes oruntil golden brown.

17. Corncakes

Ingredients:

1 ¼ c. whole wheat flour

⅓ c. cornmeal (or fresh ground popcorn kernels)

1 egg (can use food storage substitution, see chart)

⅓ c. granulated sugar

1 ½ c. buttermilk (can use food storage substitution, see chart)

1 tsp. baking powder

1 tsp. baking soda

¼ c. vegetable oil

½ tsp. salt

Directions:

Preheat a skillet over medium heat. Spray skillet with nonstick spray. Combine all ingredients in a large bowl with a mixer set on medium speed. Mix until smooth, but don't over mix. Pour the batter by ¼ – ⅓ cup portions into the hot pan and cook for 1 to 3 minutes per side or until brown. Repeat with remaining batter.

18. Cream of Chicken Soup

Ingredients:

4 T. of any white bean ground, ground into 5 T. of bean flour

1 ¾ c. water

4 tsp. chicken bouillon

Directions:

Combine all ingredients and mix well. Cook on stovetop at medium temperature until thick and boiling. The soup should boil for 3 minutes to ensure that the beans get all the way cooked for safety reasons.

19. Creamy Potato Soup

Ingredients:

4 c. cubed potatoes

½ c. minced onions (can use food storage substitution, see chart)

2 tsp. salt

3 T. chicken bouillon

2 c. diced carrots (can use food storage substitution, see chart)

2 c. diced celery (can use food storage substitution, see chart)

10 oz frozen broccoli (can use food storage substitution, see chart)

1 T. dry mustard

4 T. white bean flour mixed with ¾ c. water (any white bean ground into flour)

Cheddar cheese for topping

Directions:

In one pot cover the potatoes and onions with water, and add the chicken bouillon and salt. In a different pot (there's a reason for the 2 pots), put all the carrots, celery, and broccoli together with very little water and start. If using freeze dried veggies, add a little more water. Once the potatoes are done cooking and are soft and tender, take a masher, and very LIGHTLY mash them. This will get the soup creamy without flour, butter, and milk. After the potatoes are slightly mashed, add the carrots, celery and broccoli with the water. At this point it should be a little on the li uidy side, add the white bean flour/water mixture to thicken. Make sure you leave it boiling for at least 3 minutes

to get the beans cooked. Add the dry mustard.
Feel free to top with cheese.

20. Curried Lentils & Rice

Ingredients:

2 c. long-grain white rice

1 T. vegetable or canola oil

1 T. curry powder

½ tsp. onion powder

4 c. water

1 c. lentils (red or brown)

1 tsp. honey

1 T. balsamic vinegar

1 tsp. salt

Directions:

In one saucepan, cook rice according to
package directions. In second large saucepan,

heat oil & stir in curry powder & powdered onion. Heat the spiced oil mixture for 2 minutes while stirring. Add the 4 cups of water and lentils, stir & bring to boil. Cover and simmer for 20-25 minutes or until lentils are soft. Remove from heat and stir in the honey, balsamic vinegar & salt. Serve spooned over rice. May garnish with sour cream or salsa (if desiring a dairy-free alternative).

21. Enchilada Pie (Food Storage)

Ingredients:

1 ½ c. of cooked black beans

¼ c. dehydrated onion

1 batch of cream of chicken soup from been flour (recipe included)

4 oz can of diced green chilies

8 oz can of enchilada sauce

6 whole wheat tortillas (see Whole Wheat Tortilla recipe included)

2 c. freeze dried cheese

2 c. freeze dried chicken

Directions:

Cook tortillas and black beans. Hydrate chicken and cheese (the measurements given are the ingredients dry) While chicken and cheese is hydrating make cream of chicken bean sauce. Add beans, onions, cream of chicken sauce, diced green chilies, enchilada sauce, and chicken in a large bowl. Place tortillas in greased 9 by 13 inch pan. Top with half the bean mixture and half the cheese. Repeat the layers. Bake at 350 degrees for 40 minutes. Cool slightly and cut in s uares.

22. Enchilada Pie (Traditional Recipe)

Ingredients:

1 can of black beans

1 lg onion

1 can of cream of chicken

1 can of cream of mushroom

¾ cup of milk

4 oz can diced green chilies

8 oz can mild enchilada sauce

1 pkg soft tortillas

½ lb cheddar cheese, grated

½ lb monterrey cheese, grated

3 chicken breasts shredded

Directions:

Wash and cook beans. Mix next 6 ingredients with beans. Place tortillas in greased 9 by 13 inch pan. Top with half the bean mixture and half the cheese. Repeat the layers.

Bake at 350 degrees for 40 minutes. Cool slightly and cut in s uares.

23. Ezekiel Bread

Ingredients:

2 ½ c. wheat berries

1 ½ c. spelt flour

½ c. barley

½ c. millet

¼ c. dry green lentils

2 T. dry great northern beans

2 T. dry kidney beans

2 T. dried pinto beans

4 c. warm water

1 c. honey

½ c. olive oil

2 (¼ ounce) packages active dry yeast

2 tsp. salt

Directions:

Measure the water, honey, olive oil, and yeast into a large bowl. Let sit for 3 to 5 minutes. Stir all of the grains and beans together until well mixed. Grind in a grain mill. If you are using spelt, use ¼ c. less of the grains. If you are using spelt flour, use measurement indicated. Add fresh milled flour and salt to the yeast mixture; stir until well mixed, about 10 minutes.

The dough will be like that of a batter bread. Pour dough into two greased 9 x 5 inch loaf pans. Let rise in a warm place for about 1 hour, or until dough has reached top of the pan. Bake at 350 degrees for 45 to 50 minutes, or until loaves are golden brown.

24. Grandma Lori's Sugar Cookies

Cookie Ingredients:

2 c. butter – room temp.

2 c. white sugar

2 eggs

2 tsp. vanilla

1 c. sour cream (no light or fat free)

6 c. white flour

2 tsp. baking soda

1 tsp. salt

Frosting Ingredients:

Ingredients:

½ c. butter

8 oz. cream cheese

1 tsp. vanilla

3 c. powdered sugar

Directions:

Beat the first 4 ingredients very well, then fold in sour cream. Add flour, soda and salt.

This is uite a sticky dough, so you roll it out on a well-floured surface. Roll them a little thicker than normal cookies. Bake at 350 for 7-10 min. Do not overcook. Let cool, then place on wax paper. Frosting: Mix first 3 ingredients, then mix in powdered sugar.

25. Granola Bars

Ingredients:

4 ½ c. rolled oats

1 c. all-purpose flour (or whole wheat)

1 tsp. baking soda

1 tsp. vanilla extract

⅔ c. butter, softened

½ c. honey

⅓ c. packed brown sugar

2 c. miniature semisweet chocolate chips

Directions:

Lightly grease one 9×13 inch pan. In a large mixing bowl combine the oats, flour, baking soda, vanilla, butter or margarine, honey and brown sugar. Stir in the 2 cups assorted chocolate chips. Lightly press mixture into the prepared pan. Bake at 325 degrees for 18 to 22 minutes or until golden brown. Let cool for 10 minutes then cut into bars. Let bars cool completely in pan before removing or serving.

26. Greek Lentil Soup

Ingredients:

2 c. lentils, dried

4 c. cold water

1 c. onion,

1 clove garlic, crushed

4 c. beef broth

¼ tsp. black pepper

½ c. celery, chopped (can use food storage substitution, see chart)

2 c. tomatoes, stewed

1 bay leaf

1 c. carrots (can use food storage substitution, see chart)

3 T. parsley, chopped (can use food storage substitution, see chart)

½ tsp. oregano (can use food storage substitution, see chart)

2 T. vinegar

Directions:

Wash lentils, drain well. Combine lentils with all ingredients except vinegar. Bring to a boil.

Lower heat; cover and simmer 2 hours or until lentils are tender. Add vinegar and simmer 30 minutes more. Remove bay leaf. Serve soup.

27. Homemade Egg McMuffins

Instructions:

1 egg

1 T. egg white powder (e uivalent to 3 egg whites)

2 T. water

Directions:

Mix and scramble egg, egg white powder, and water. Fry in pan. Use as the base for an Egg McMuffin by adding ham and cheese and putting on an English Muffin. It tastes the same as using free egg whites, but you don't waste as many yolks and you can still cut back on the fat and calories.

28. Homemade Hummus

Ingredients:

2 c. soaked chickpeas or 1 can beans, drained

¼ c. lemon juice

1 T. tahini (sesame seed oil)

2 cloves garlic or 2 tsp. garlic powder

1 tsp. curry powder

½ jar of roasted red peppers, drained

Directions:

Mince the garlic, put in food processor. Add the garbanzo beans, puree. Add the oil and juice, puree again. Drain and add roasted red peppers, add curry, blend.

If the beans are soft, then you'll only have to process for a minute. When using soaked, but not cooked beans, process for five minutes or until smooth. Use as a spread or a dip.

29. Homemade Mayonnaise

Ingredients:

1 T. powdered egg (heaping)

1 T. water

1 pinch of sugar

½ tsp. salt

1 T. lemon juice

½ tsp. mustard (any flavor you enjoy)

½ - ¾ c. oil

Directions:

Mix all the ingredients except the oil in a small blender, food processor, or in a bowl with a hand wand style blender. Add a few drops of oil and mix until well blended. Add a few more drops and mix until well blended. Keep adding drops very slowly with full mixing in between until mayonnaise thickens up. This recipe makes a small batch as it only stores in the fridge 3-5 days. You can double or triple the recipe if you need more.

30. Homemade Pasta

Ingredients:

1 ½ c. semolina flour

1 ½ c. freshly ground whole wheat flour

½ tsp. salt

4 eggs

¼ c. water

¼ c. olive oil

Directions:

Combine semolina, wheat flour, and salt. Beat eggs lightly. Mix eggs, water and oil. Stir in to four mixture until a stiff dough forms. You may need to add a little more flour.

Knead 10 minutes or until elastic. Let rest, covered for 20 minutes. Roll out thinly. Cut into desired shape or shape with machine. Cook in boiling, salted water for 2-5 minutes.

31. Homemade Ranch Dip or Dressing

Ingredients:

1 c. plain greek yogurt (full fat)

½ c. sour cream (can use food storage substitution, see chart)

½ tsp. garlic powder

½ tsp. dill

¼ tsp. pepper

3 T. minced fresh parsley (can use food storage substitution, see chart)

2 T. minced fresh chives (can use food storage substitution, see chart)

salt to taste

Directions:

Combine ingredients, and chill before serving. If you are using powdered sour cream, add ½ c. sour cream powder to the mixture, then add water slowly until you get desired texture.

32. Homemade Rice-A-Roni

Ingredients:

2 c. rice

1 c. angel hair, vermicelli or spaghettini pasta, broken into very small pieces

¼ c. parsley (can use food storage substitution, see chart)

6 T. chicken bouillon powder

2 tsp. onion powder

½ tsp. garlic powder

¼ tsp. thyme

Directions:

Combine all ingredients and mix well. To prepare: Melt 2 T. butter in a skillet. Add 1 c. of the mix and stir. Add 2 ¼ c, water. Bring to a boil. Reduce heat to low, cover and simmer for 15 minutes.

33. Homemade Smoothies

Ingredients:

¾ c. of frozen strawberries (can use food storage substitution, see chart)

½ c. of frozen blueberries (can use food storage substitution, see chart)

½ c. of frozen peaches or raspberries (can use food storage substitution, see chart)

1 c. of powdered milk prepared

½ c. yogurt (frozen works great)

Some of sugar if you think it needs it

Directions:

Pour milk into blender. Add fruit, yogurt, and any other sweetener you desire.

34. Honey Whole Wheat Bread

Ingredients:

2 c. all-purpose flour

1 tsp. salt

1 pkg.   uick rise yeast

¾ c. milk (can use food storage substitution, see chart)

¾ c. water

2 T. honey

2 T. vegetable oil

2 c. whole wheat flour

Directions:

Combine 1 ½ cups all-purpose flour, salt, and yeast in large mixing bowl. Heat milk, water, honey and oil until hot to touch. Gradually add to dry ingredients. Beat 2 minutes at medium speed of mixer, scraping bowl occasionally. Add ½ cup all-purpose flour.

Beat at high speed for 2 minutes, scraping bowl occasionally. With spoon, stir in whole wheat flour and enough additional all-purpose flour to make stiff dough. Knead on lightly floured surface until smooth and elastic, about 6-8 minutes. Place in greased bowl, turning to grease top. Cover, let rest for 10 minutes. Spray loaf pan with vegetable pan spray. Roll dough to 12×8" rectangle. Roll up from short end to make loaf. Pinch seam and ends to seal. Place, seam side down, in prepared pan. Cover, let rise in warm place until doubled in size, about 30 minutes. Bake at 375° for 35 minutes or until bread sounds hollow when tapped. Remove from pan, cool in a wire rack.

35. Hot Fudge Sauce

Ingredients:

1 can evaporated milk (can use food storage substitution, see chart)

2 c. semisweet chocolate chips

½ c. sugar

1 T. butter or margarine (spreads with at least 65% vegetable oil)

1 tsp. vanilla

Directions:

In a 2- uart sauce pan mix your evaporated milk with a whisk. Add chocolate chips and sugar and heat over MEDIUM heat, stirring constantly until it boils. Remove from heat and stir in butter and vanilla. Let cool for at least 30 minutes or until sauce begins to thicken. Serve warm. Store your remaining sauce covered in the refrigerator up to 4 weeks. Sauce become firm when refrigerated; heat slightly before serving (sauce will become thin if overheated).

*Recipe from Everyday Food Storage

36. Meatballs Tetrazzini

Ingredients:

1 batch of basic meatballs (see Basic Meatball recipe)

8 oz package spaghetti

1 can condensed tomato soup

¼ c. freeze dried onion

½ tsp. salt

1 c. milk

⅛ tsp. pepper

8 oz shredded cheddar cheese (can use food storage substitution, see chart)

Directions:

Prepare basic meatball recipe. Preheat oven to 350 degrees. Cook spaghetti and drain. Combine soup, milk, onion, salt, pepper, and cheese. Head until cheese is melted. Arrange meatballs and spaghetti in a 9×13 pan. Pour li uid mixture over meatballs and toss to mix well. Back for 30 minutes until hot and serve immediately.

37. Mexican Casserole

Ingredients:

1 family size package Kraft macaroni and cheese

(or 3 c. macaroni, ½ c. powdered cheese, 6 tsp. butter, 6 tsp. of powdered milk)

½ lb. lean hamburger browned (can use food storage substitution, see chart)

½ onion, chopped (can use food storage substitution, see chart)

1 can chili with beans

1 can tomato soup

1 T. chili powder

1 can corn

Cheddar cheese, cubed (optional)

Fritos (optional)

Directions:

Preheat oven to 350º. Cook Kraft dinner according to directions in large pot. Meanwhile, brown hamburger with onion. Add to Kraft dinner with remaining ingredients. Heat through. Pour into casserole dish and top with Fritos. Cover and bake 30 minutes.

38. No-Bake Peanut Butter Energy Bites

Ingredients:

2 c. old fashion oats

½ c. peanut butter

⅓ c. raw honey

½ c. of chocolate

1 tsp. vanilla

Directions:

Put all the ingredients in a bowl and mix. Put the mixture in the fridge for 30 minutes to cool. After the mixture is cool, roll into balls. Store in an airtight container in the fridge or freezer.

39. Patriotic Jello

Ingredients:

2 3 oz packages blue jello

2 3 oz packages strawberry jello

2 envelopes unflavored gelatin

14 oz can sweetened condensed Milk (can use food storage substitution, see chart)

Freeze-dried strawberries (can use food storage substitution, see chart)

Freeze-ried blueberries (can use food storage substitution, see chart)

Spiff-E-Whip

Directions:

Make your blue layer of jello. Mix 2 packages of blue jello with 2 cups of boiling water until dissolved. Then add 1 cup of ice cold water and stir. Pour into a 9×12 pan. Sprinkle freeze-dried blueberries evenly into the pan and stir them in so they are covered with li uid. Let set in fridge for 4 hours or overnight.

Make your white layer of jello. Sprinkle 2 envelopes of unflavored gelatin into ½ a cup of cold water. After it thickens, add 1 ½ cups of boiling water and mix in until it dissolves.

Stir in the can of sweetened condensed milk until smooth. Let cool (but don't leave it out too long) Pour over hardened blue layer. Let chill for 4 hours or overnight.

Make your red layer of jello. Mix 2 packages of blue jello with 2 cups of boiling water until dissolved. Then add 1 cup of ice cold water and stir. Sprinkle freeze-dried strawberries into the li uid. Pour entire mixture over top of white layer. Let set in fridge for 4 hours or overnight. Once the red layer has set firmly, you can decorate the top with a flag if desired. Mix 1 cup of Spiff-E-Whip with 1 cup of ice water and beat with a mixer for about 3-4 minutes until it has a whipped cream consistency.

While beating the whipped cream, reconstitute some freeze-dried blueberries and strawberries for the topping. Spread the whipped cream over top and decorate like a flag.

www.ingramcontent.com/pod-product-compliance
Lightning Source LLC
Chambersburg PA
CBHW071602270726

48661CB00017B/349